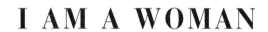

I AM A WOMAN

I AM A WOMAN

Your highest calling

Jo Wyse

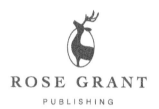

ROSE GRANT

PUBLISHING

First published 2016 by Rose Grant Publishing
Designed by Sarah Anderson
Copyright © 2016 Rose Grant Publishing
85 Killams Green, Taunton, Somerset TA1 3YQ
United Kingdom

For my daughter,
whom I am yet to meet...

About Jo

Jo Wyse is a writer, publisher and broadcaster who worked
as a presenter on BBC and commercial radio for over 15 years.

After meeting her partner Austin in 2007, Jo left her job in mainstream
media to pursue her passion of communicating 'new-thinking' messages
about health, well-being and the power of human consciousness.

Visit www.thewysecentre.co.uk for more books,
mp3s & radio programmes

Acknowledgements

So much of this book was inspired by the writings and teachings
of Dr Christine Page. For more information about her work
please visit www.christinepage.com

Thank you Christine for teaching me and so many other women
and girls what it really means to be feminine.

I would also like to thank the masculine in my life, Austin,
my protector who saw the woman in me when I couldn't.

Table of Contents

"To be feminine is
to become passive,
to be feminine
is to allow;
to be feminine is
to wait,
to be feminine is
not to be in a hurry
and tense;
to be feminine
is to be in love."

- Osho

Introduction

This book is for women curious about how powerful their bodies really are.

This book is for women who have painful cycles, irregular cycles or no cycles at all. Women who have been diagnosed with conditions of their reproductive organs or even had some or all of those areas removed. Women who have had those sacred parts of themselves mistreated or abused. Women who have had babies, women who are unable to have babies, women who don't want to have babies, women who haven't yet had babies. Women who have gone through or are going through the menopause and girls who are about to become women.

Whatever stage of womanhood you have reached and whatever the relationship you have with your cycle... this book is for you.

It may well be that your body isn't in tune with the rhythms of nature that this book describes and that is okay too, because there is never just one cycle; there are cycles within cycles. Your only job here is to become aware of how powerful your body is and to use this knowledge in a way that works for you.

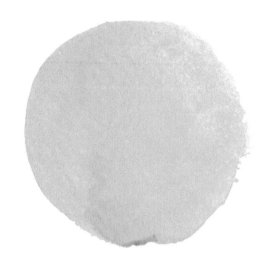

"The greatest thing you'll
ever learn is just to love,
and be loved in return."

- Eden Ahbez

I Am Love

You are here to learn, to expand and grow in love...
so that The Great Mother in turn can learn,
expand and grow in love.

"Amidst the worldly comings and goings, observe how endings become beginnings."

- The Tao Te Ching

I Am Cyclical

Long before watches and clocks existed, our ancestors experienced
the passage of time by observing cycles; they watched the birth, growth,
decay and death of all living things, of all of nature, and they acknowledged
and celebrated the significance and the sacredness of each
of the four stages.

They saw the four stages in each and every day, in each and every season,
in the movement of the stars, the planets and the heavens. They understood
that even their own breath was part of an ever-decreasing
and ever-increasing cycle.

A cycle of birth, growth, decay and death.

"Let life be as beautiful
as summer flowers and
death be as beautiful
as autumn leaves."

- Rabindranath Tagore

I Am a Reminder of a Solemn Promise

Our ancestors believed in a covenant, a solemn promise, an agreement with The Great Mother that she would constantly provide them with inspiration to birth new life and ideas so that they could manifest, create and grow, but that when the time came for those creations to decay and die they would not only release them... they would offer everything they didn't need from each cycle back to her as new seeds of consciousness so that a more expanded, more loving cycle could be born again.

A woman's body is a constant reminder of that covenant, that she is here to consciously birth new life so that those creations can grow, decay and eventually die in their own way and in their own time.

"The wiser the woman,
the wiser everything
is around her."

I Am an Alchemic Vessel

You may have been told that the only reason women have cycles is to have babies, and while that is part of the story, it isn't the whole story. You see an average woman in her lifetime will have hundreds and hundreds of cycles, yet will only give birth to one or two children, so what is the purpose of the remaining cycles?

Well the purpose of a woman's cycle is not only to birth babies but also to birth new ideas and new levels of consciousness; that's right, the eggs in her body represent the potential for a baby but they also represent the potential for bringing any creation to life.

A woman's body is an alchemic vessel that has the power to transform a few cells into a human life form and an invisible thought into a physical reality. Becoming in tune with and honouring the birth, growth, decay and death stages brings meaning and purpose to her creations and helps her and everything around her to expand in consciousness.

"The deeper that sorrow
carves into your being,
the more joy you
can contain."

- Kahil Gibran

I Am Joy and Sorrow

However, over time, not only has humanity lost touch with the concept of cycling, the decay and death stages have become processes to fear.

This is because birth and growth are exciting times that fill us with hope and optimism, but decay and death can be sad times that bring despair and unhappiness.

Yet it is impossible to have night without day or positive without negative... as the prophet Kahil Gibran once said 'the deeper that sorrow carves into your being, the more joy you can contain.'

A woman honours all stages of the cycle.

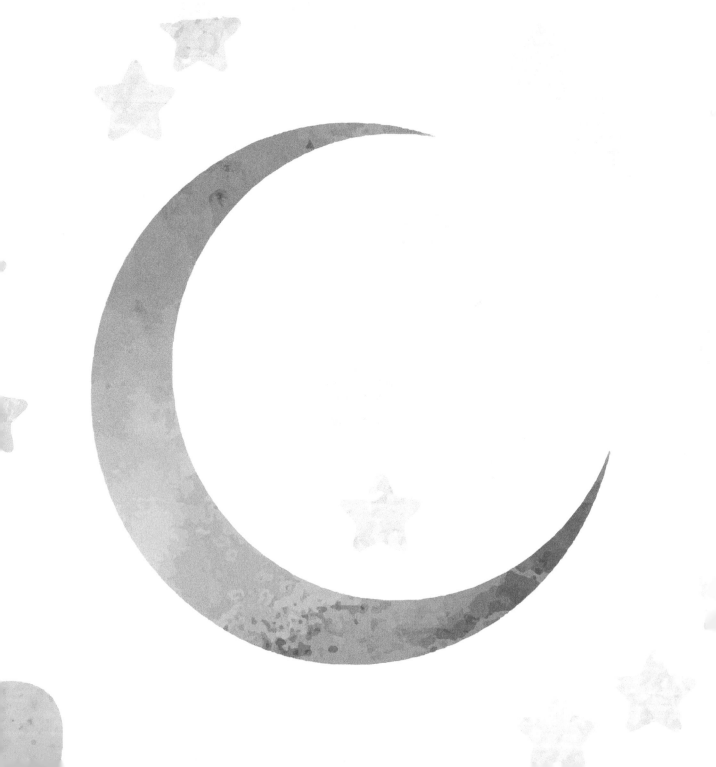

I Am a Mirror of the Moon

As above, so below...

Observing the moon can offer great insight because the waxing,
waning, fullness, darkness and the length of the lunar cycles
are all said to mirror the menstrual cycle.

Our ancestral sisters knew this and would synchronise with each other's
cycles and the lunar cycles to obtain maximum wisdom during each
of the four main stages.

I Am The Crone

On a new moon, they would gather to share stories and they understood
that their bleeding symbolised a cleansing of any redundant emotions that
they (or members of their family) had experienced since their last cycle.

This was a time when they were at their wisest,
and it was a time for letting go.

This new moon is the Death stage, the Winter stage,
the stage of The Crone.

I Am The Virgin

When the moon began to wax and moved into its first quarter, the women,
having released what they no longer needed, would have increased their
conscious awareness; they had a renewed sense of clarity
and were ready and open to learning again.

The waxing moon is the Birth stage, the Spring stage,
the stage of The Virgin.

I Am The Mother

When the moon became full, when it could be seen in all its glory in the
night sky, the women would ovulate and be at the height of their creativity.

They would be wonderful communicators, expressive and outgoing, and
they would feel emotionally and sexually connected, keen to obtain
and nurture new seeds of consciousness.

The full moon is the Growth stage, the Summer stage,
the stage of The Mother.

I Am The Enchantress

…and when the moon began to wane and moved to its third quarter, the women would become introspective and reflective about what may need to be harvested and what may need to be released from this cycle.

The women at this time were at the height of their intuition and assertiveness.

The waning moon is the Decay stage, the Autumn stage, the stage of The Enchantress.

"A woman's highest calling
is to lead a man back to
his soul so as to unite
him with Source...
A man's highest calling
is to protect a woman
so she is free to walk the
earth unharmed."

- Cherokee proverb

I Am Leading The Way

A native American teacher once said that a thousand years of peace will
come when women (not men) have healed their hearts... and women
have been given an innate power to do that by...

Honouring the birth, growth, decay and death stages of their cycles, using
the waxing, waning, fullness and darkness of the moon as their guide.

Cleansing their redundant emotions and the redundant emotions
of their family through monthly bleeding and rituals.

Realising and utilising the ability they have to not only birth babies
but also to birth ideas with new levels of consciousness.

"A woman's highest calling is to lead a man back
to his soul so as to unite him with Source...
A man's highest calling is to protect a woman
so she is free to walk the earth unharmed."
- Cherokee proverb

Lightning Source UK Ltd.
Milton Keynes UK
UKOW07n1513280617
304193UK00003B/6/P